I0429552

Omega-3 Made Easy: The Ultimate Guide To Understanding, Using, And Benefiting From Omega 3

All rights Reserved. No part of this publication or the information in it may be quoted from or reproduced in any form by means such as printing, scanning, photocopying or otherwise without prior written permission of the copyright holder.

Disclaimer and Terms of Use: Effort has been made to ensure that the information in this book is accurate and complete, however, the author and the publisher do not warrant the accuracy of the information, text and graphics contained within the book due to the rapidly changing nature of science, research, known and unknown facts and internet. The Author and the publisher do not hold any responsibility for errors, omissions or contrary interpretation of the subject matter herein. This book is presented solely for motivational and informational purposes only.

Table of Contents

Introduction

Omega-3 fatty acids are one of the very popular types of fats that is getting all the attention these days. This is a unique type of fat that has loads and loads of health benefits. This is the reason why you see a lot of television commercials, radio advertisements and many of the food products emphasize on the omega 3 fatty acids. Any diet supplement that you find in the market will now be containing omega 3 as its main constituent. But, there are also a lot of foods in the form of vegetables, fruits and meat that contains more amounts of omega 3 fatty acids. If you would like to maintain a healthy body and a healthy heart, then you need to think of going for foods that contain rich sources of omega 3 fatty acids. This fat belongs to the polyunsaturated fatty acid group of fats, which is normally denoted as PUFA.

A lot of nutritionists and medical practitioners now regard omega 3 and omega 6 fatty acids as the most essential fats. It is a must for the human body as it performs a lot of body functions right from building of healthy body cells to maintaining the performance of nerve and brain functions. Omega 3 fatty acids cannot be produced by our body and this can only be got from the food that we consume.

Types Of Omega 3 Fatty Acids

There are three common types of omega 3 fatty acids that are very important for maintaining a healthy body. They are ALA, EPA and DHA. ALA or alpha-linolenic acid is one of the simplest forms of omega - 3. The ALA must be an important and integral part of your diet as your body cannot produce the ALA. You need to take in ALA rich foods to maintain a healthy body. Some of the more commonly eaten plant and animal foods contain ALA. Hence, getting adequate amounts of alpha-linolenic-acid that is required for the body will not be a problem at all. The other omega-3s are more complicated than the ALA as it contains more double bonds. Your body has the capacity to take in the ALAs and transform it into other omega-3s.

The EPA (eicosapentaenoic acid) has five double bonds and the DHA (docosahexaenoic acid) has six double bonds. It has been researched and found out that EPA and DHA offers more and better health benefits than ALA. These two types of Omega-3 fatty acids help in reducing the risk of many chronic health diseases and also support a lot of the body systems. So, if you need to stay healthy, then you need to take in adequate amounts of omega-3s, in particular ALA,

DHA and EPA. You should consume ALA containing foods on a daily basis and believe that your body can make all the EPA and DHA needed by your body from the ALA rich foods that you are consuming. It would be ideal for you to extract the needed EPA and DHA right from the food that you eat.

Foods To Eat

If you are a strict veggie and do not want to include any of the animal foods, including cheese, milk and eggs in your diet, then you need to make sure that you consume a lot of sea plants or some fermented foods to produce the required amount of DHA. But, the option to include DHA rich foods are limited for a strict veggie as it is totally absent in land plants. A person who is generally vegetarian, but has the habit of eating fish along with his or her veggie diet will find ALA rich foods in plants and of course fish and can find the EPA and DHA rich foods in cheese, eggs, milk, yoghurt and in a few land plants. A person who eats a vegetarian diet that also includes cheese, eggs, yoghurt and milk will get adequate amount of ALA and get a limited amount of DHA and EPA from land plant foods that are fermented with the help of a certain fungi. If you are a person who eats plant food as well as meat, then you get enough amounts of ALA, EPA and DHA from many plants as well as from many meats of grass eating animals. You need to make a lot of adjustments to your diet if you want to include foods that are rich in DHA and EPA in your daily diet.

A person who is very healthy should eat ALA rich foods like walnut, flax seeds, tofu and spinach every day. As they have a healthy body, they can rely on their bodies to convert ALA into DHA and EPA. But, it is still not completely proven and researched that a person will be able to actively convert the required amount of DHA and EPA from the ALA containing foods that he or she takes in every day. It is recommended that people who do not take in animal foods, including milk or cheese, must consult their health practitioner to find out the right supplementation of omega-3 fatty acids that they should consume. If you are a person who avoids sea foods, but takes in animal foods, then you should be always looking to consume animal foods that are rich in omega-3s as this will help you to get the required amount of DHA and EPA that your body needs. If you stick on to a diet of taking in the fish for three times a week, then you will be able to bring in adequate levels of EPA and DHA in your meal plan easily. Consuming fish regularly or at least two to three servings per week will offer you the required amounts of omega-3 fatty acids that will help in preventing any cardiovascular diseases as well as offer other health benefits.

ALAs Role In Health Support

The following are some of the different roles that ALA or alpha-linolenic acid plays in supporting your health.

- ALA can be used by your body to produce energy for your body cells and is used for energy purposes by the body.

- ALA is the main building block for EPA and DHA and without ALA and its by-products, DHA and EPA, your immune system, cardiovascular system, inflammatory system and nervous system will not function properly.

- As much as 85% of the dietary ALA is used by your body as an energy source and the remaining 15 percent of the dietary ALA is used to prepare omega-3 fats DHA and EPA, which helps in the overall health of the body.

The following are the foods that are rich in alpha-linolenic acid or ALA:

- Flax seeds

- Walnuts

- Avocados

- Vegetables like kale, turnip greens, collard, spinach, green beans, Brussels sprouts, lettuce, summer and winter squash

- Fishes like tuna, shrimp, halibut, cod and scallops, sardines and salmon

- Mustard seeds

- Strawberries

- Raspberries

- Legumes like soybeans, miso and tofu

- Plant oils like canola oil and soy oil

The most commonly consumed animal foods like beef and eggs are also said to contain varying amounts of ALA. Cereal based foods, vegetables and beans are some of the foods that people eat very commonly and all these foods are found to contain small traces of nutritionally relevant ALA.

EPAs Role In Health Support

The following are the ways in which consumption of adequate amounts of EPA or eicosapentaenoic acid will help you to maintain your body.

- If you have adequate amounts of EPA in your body, then it will ensure that your inflammatory system performs and function properly. Prostaglandins are the main messaging molecule in the inflammatory system and it is made directly from the EPA.

- EPA will take care of excessive inflammation as well as inflammation related diseases that target your body. It will help in lowering the inflammations that spring up on your body.

- The prostaglandins developed from omega-3 fatty acids will play an important role in weakening the inflammations and will also help in balancing out the pro-inflammatory effect caused by omega-6 fats.

DHAs Role In Health Support

The following are the roles that DHA or docosahexaenoic acid performs to ensure proper functioning of the body.

- It will help in proper functioning of the nervous system and ensures that the brain also functions properly.

- DHA accounts for 9 to 12 percent of the total weight of the brain and abut 15 to 20 percent of the fat I the brain is represented by DHA.

- If there is a drop in the DHA levels in the brain, then it is found to slow the neurological development in children and is also associated with cognitive impairment.

- Deficiency in DHA is found to cause a wide variety of nervous disorders like: Parkinson's disease, severe multiple sclerosis as well as reducing the reasoning ability in children.

Foods Rich In DHA And EPA

One of the best sources of EPA and DHA are fish. The cold water fishes are in fact the best dietary sources of DHA and EPA. Salmons, cod and sardines are having rich sources of omega 3 fatty acids and they are very rich in EPA and DHA. You can gain up to 2 to 4 grams of omega-3 fatty acid content from these fishes for every 100 grams that you consume. This will help in the overall functioning of your body, especially your heart. High concentrations of DHA are found to be very common in salmons. These fishes do not prepare their own EPA and DHA and they get it from the sea plants that they feed on. More amounts of EPA and DHA can be got from these fishes rather than from taking in the sea plant weeds as the fishes store these nutrients in their cells. Farmed fish like catfish and tilapia are also good sources of EPA and DHA. Land animal meats are also a good source for EPA and DHA, but they do not contain as much of the omega -3 fatty acids that you get in sea water fishes. It is ideal for you to eat meat of land animals that eat grass. Cows and chicken are also good sources of omega -3s and the milk and the eggs that they produce are also good sources of omega -3s. An egg can sometimes even contain about 350 mgs of omega-3 fats. Grass fed cows can give up to 150 mgs of omega-3s in an 8 ounce cup of milk. DHA is more commonly found in the eggs and milk than the EPA. Some of the fortified foods that you can buy in the market like: juices, snack foods and margarine spreads are also rich in omega-3s.

Omega-3 fatty acids are a mix of polyunsaturated fatty acids, docosahexanoic acid (DHA)(found in fish), eicosapentaenic acid (EPA) and alpha-linolenic acid (ALA) (found in plants). These polyunsaturated fats help to lower cholesterol levels and reduce the inflammation of the body. Our body does not produce these fatty acids and hence it is necessary to get the omega 3 fatty acids from our diet or through supplements. There are many health benefits that you can get from daily consumption of omega 3 fatty acids.

1. Increases HDL Cholesterol Levels

Studies have shown that fishes, walnuts and fish oil as well as omega-3 supplements can decrease triglyceride levels. You need to take at least two to three servings of fatty fish like sardines, cods and salmons a week to enjoy increased good HDL cholesterol levels and to lower bad triglycerides.

2. Switch To Unsaturated Oils

It is high time that you switched to unsaturated fats rather than using saturated fats like butter, cream and so that are derived from animal sources. These animal fats are said to contain high levels of LDL (bad cholesterol) which will result in clogging your arteries after some time. This might also lead to heart attacks and heart failure. You can easily prevent this by switching over to unsaturated fats and oils that are derived from fishes or nuts. They will help in lowering the cholesterol levels and thereby maintain a healthy heart. Some of the most common changes that you can make in your day to day diet are:

- Using olive oil as a dressing and flavoring agent on your vegetable salads

- Using canola oil or other vegetate oil for sautéing purposes instead of butter

- Spreading olive oil on your bread instead of using butter

- Replace your fat rich butter with non-hydrogenated margarine

- Prepare creamy sauces with low fat yoghurt instead of using rich cream

3. Builds Bone Strength

It has been researched that people who take adequate amounts of omega-3s on a daily basis help in increasing the calcium levels in the body. This will ensure that the bone strength is increased. People who do not eat sufficient amounts of fatty acids that contain EPA, GLA and DHA have lesser bone strength and density than people who take in normal recommended levels of fatty acids.

4. Include Nuts To Your Daily Menu

Nuts are rich sources of omega 3 and omega 6 fatty acids. It helps in preventing heart diseases and this is the reason why it is recommended to eat a handful of nuts every day. Nuts are the ideal snack that you can think of having between breakfast and lunch. It is also a healthy snack when compared to other fat-rich oily snacks. Some of the different ways that you can prepare the nuts to add taste to your daily menu:

- Add toasted almonds to your baked chicken dish to increase the taste of the chicken

- You can garnish your salads with walnuts to add crunchy taste to your salads.

- Eat stir fries with almonds or cashews

5. Reduces Cancer Risk

Omega 3 fatty acid diet is found to be very helpful in preventing as well as reducing the risk caused by colon cancer. Women who take adequate amounts of omega 3 fatty acids foods in their diet will find that they are less likely prone to diseases such as breast cancer and prostate cancer. A low fat diet that is rich in omega-3 fatty acids from fish or fish oil is ideal in preventing the progress of prostate cancer.

6. Lowers Depression Levels

Fish oil is a rich source of omega-3 fatty acids and it helps in reducing the depression levels. People eating foods that contain higher levels of omega-3s are found to enjoy reduced mood swings and also enjoy an increase in the effects of antidepressants. It has also been found out that the omega-3 fatty acids helps in increasing your memory power as well as helping the nervous system to perform properly. It is a powerful source that helps fight depression. People who are suffering from bipolar disorder will be able to easily fight depression and other mental problems if they regularly take in omega 3 fatty acids. Omega-3s are also found to reduce depression and maniac problems in juvenile bipolar disorder. It is highly effective to treat women experiencing postpartum depression. The supplementation of fatty acids also helps in reducing attention-deficit/hyperactivity disorder (ADHD) in children.

7. Controls Diabetes

It has been researched that eating fatty fish that is rich in omega 3 fatty acids has positive effects on blood sugar levels in people with diabetes. Regular consumption of omega-3 rich foods, especially fish helps diabetes people to lower fasting glucose concentration and also helps in increasing insulin levels significantly. It is also found out that eating fish rich in omega 3 fatty acids reduce the development of type-2 diabetes. Taking in omega 3 fatty acid supplements regularly resulted in reducing homocysteine levels in patients suffering from diabetes. It will also help in improving the micro and macro-vascular functions with respect to type-2 diabetes mellitus. Taking in fish oil and long chain omega 3 fatty acid foods reduces the risk of total mortality associated with coronary heart diseases in women suffering from diabetes.

8. Controls Physiological Functions

Omega 3 fatty acids are found to play a very vital role in the development of prostaglandins. This will in turn help in taking care and regulating all the important physiological functions of the body. It will help in controlling blood pressure levels, better nerve transmission, preventing blood clotting and also takes care of allergic responses.

9. Fights Dementia and Alzheimer's

If you do not take adequate amounts of omega 3 fatty acids in your diet, then you are likely to see an increase in the risk of catching dementia. It has been researched and proved by scientists that person who takes adequate amounts of omega 3 fatty acid foods that are particularly rich in DHA have been found to be safe from dementia and Alzheimer's disease. Consuming fatty fish rich in DHA at least twice a week will decrease the risk of catching Alzheimer's disease and dementia. Regular consumption of omega 3 fatty acids was found to be very effective in treating children with autism. Taking in omega-3s along with required quantities of zinc and magnesium proved to be beneficial for treating emotional, attentional and behavioral problems in children as well as adolescents.

10.   Reduces Child Asthma Risk

One of the ways to decrease the risk of developing asthma is to eat a lot of omega-3 fatty acids. You need to eat a lot of fishes that are rich in omega 3 fatty acids to decrease the risk of getting asthma. It has been proved that children who ate fatty fish are less likely to develop asthma throughout their life cycle. The risk of wheezing was found to be reduced by about 36 percent in children who consumed fatty fish regularly between the ages of six months to one year. Adults also can enjoy the benefits of omega 3 rich fatty fish that helps in reducing asthma symptoms and problems.

11. Lowering Heart Diseases

The fish oils are rich in omega -3 fatty acids like EPA and DHA and are found to reduce the level of triglycerides in our body. Having elevated triglyceride levels is a reason for heart diseases. Consuming fatty fish regularly, at least thrice a week will help in getting two important forms of omega 3 fatty acids, called eicosapentaenoic acid (EPA) and docosahexaenoic acid (DHA). These fatty acids will help in reducing the inflammation and thereby prevent heart diseases. People who are suffering from coronary heart diseases are advised to take more quantities of fatty fish to prevent artery blockage and blood clotting. You should be going for a diet that is low in saturated fat and rich in monounsaturated and polyunsaturated fats to prevent heart diseases. Fish oil has been shown to reduce the problems of irregular heartbeats or arrhythmias. It is very effective in reducing the risk of stroke and also helps in effectively treating the narrowing and hardening of the arteries.

- If you take fish oil supplements regularly after you have had a first heart attack, then the risk of getting another heart attack is greatly reduced.

- It will also help in reducing total mortality and sudden death in patients who have a history of heart diseases.

- It will also help in preventing atrial fibrillation in men and women who have undergone coronary artery bypass surgery.

- DHA rich omega 3 fatty acids will help in reducing the risk of peripheral arterial disease that is associated with chain smokers.

- Taking foods that are rich in higher concentrations of EPA and DHA reduces the risk of nonfatal myocardial infarction in women.

- Consumption of fatty fish will help in reducing the chances of stroke in elderly people.

- Fish oil improves endothelial function in peripheral arterial diseases and also has a amazing effect on blood viscosity for the people who suffering from peripheral vascular disease.

- The Omega-3 fatty acid that is rich in docosapentaenoic acid (DPA) will help in reducing the risk involved in peripheral arterial disease seen in smokers.

12. Reduces Symptoms Of Rheumatoid Arthritis

Omega 3 fatty acids are highly effective in reducing the stiffness and joint pains. Hence, they are good for people suffering from Rheumatoid Arthritis. Omega -3 is also found to enhance the effectiveness of anti-inflammatory drugs. The fish oil supplements that contain rich amounts of EPA and DHA help in reducing stiffness of the body as well as reduce joint pains to a great extent. Omega 3 fish oil helps in greatly reducing the severity of systemic lupus erythmeatosus symptoms.

13.   Preventing Cancer

Taking dietary foods that contain rich amounts of EPA and DHA inhibits the development of breast cancer in women and also reduces metastasis. Consumption of fatty fish will help in reducing prostate cancer specific mortality by over 60%. Omega-3s are said to have a protective effect against bacterial colonization in cystic fibrosis. It also reduces inflammations in patients suffering from cystic fibrosis.

www.ingramcontent.com/pod-product-compliance
Lightning Source LLC
Chambersburg PA
CBHW072016280526
45788CB00005B/2068